W9-DBH-311

DOES TELEVISION MAKE YOU FAT?

LIFESTYLE AND OBESITY

OBESITY & KIDS

DOES TELEVISION MAKE YOU FAT?

LIFESTYLE AND OBESITY

BY RAE SIMONS

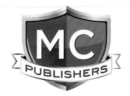

Mason Crest Publishers

MASON CREST PUBLISHERS INC.
370 Reed Road
Broomall, Pennsylvania 19008
(866)MCP-BOOK (toll free)
www.masoncrest.com

First Printing
9 8 7 6 5 4 3 2 1

Library of Congress Cataloging-in-Publication Data

Simons, Rae, 1957–
 Does television make you fat? : lifestyle and obesity / by Rae Simons.
    p. cm. — (Obesity & kids)
 Includes index.
  ISBN 978-1-4222-1712-2 (hardcover)   ISBN 978-1-4222-1705-4 (hardcover series)
  ISBN 978-1-4222-1900-3 (pbk.)   ISBN 978-1-4222-1893-8 (pbk series)
 1. Obesity—Treatment. 2. Lifestyles—Health aspects. 3. Obesity—therapy. 4. Health behavior.
 5. Exercise. I. Title.
 RC628.S6217 2010
 362.196'398—dc22
                              2010022849

Design by MK Bassett-Harvey and Wendy Arakawa.
Produced by Harding House Publishing Service, Inc.
www.hardinghousepages.com
Cover design by Torque Advertising and Design.
Printed in USA by Bang Printing.

The creators of this book have made every effort to provide accurate information, but it should not be used as a substitute for the help and services of trained professionals.

CONTENTS

INTRODUCTION
FOR THE TEACHERS

We as a society often reserve our harshest criticism for those conditions we understand the least. Such is the case for obesity. Obesity is a chronic and often-fatal disease that accounts for 400,000 deaths each year. It is second only to smoking as a cause of premature death in the United States. People suffering from obesity need understanding, support, and medical assistance. Yet what they often receive is scorn.

Today, children are the fastest growing segment of the obese population in the United States. This constitutes a public health crisis of enormous proportions. Living with childhood obesity affects self-esteem, which down the road can affect employment and attainment of higher education. But childhood obesity is much more than a social stigma. It has serious health consequences.

Childhood obesity increases the risk for poor health in adulthood—but also even during childhood. Depression, diabetes, asthma, gallstones, orthopedic diseases, and other obesity-related conditions are all on the rise in children. Recent estimates suggest that 30 to 50 percent of children born in 2000 will develop type 2 diabetes mellitus, a leading cause of preventable blindness, kidney failure, heart disease, stroke, and amputations. Obesity is undoubtedly the most pressing nutritional disorder among young people today.

If we are to reverse obesity's current trend, there must be family, community, and national objectives promoting healthy eating and exercise. As a nation, we must demand broad-based public-health initiatives to limit TV watching, curtail junk food advertising toward children, and promote physical activity. More than rhetoric, these need to be our rallying cry. Anything short of this will eventually fail, and within our lifetime obesity will become the leading cause of death in the United States if not in the world. This series is an excellent first step in battling the obesity crisis by educating young children about the risks, the realities, and what they can do to build healthy lifestyles right now.

CHAPTER 1
A DANGEROUS LIFESTYLE

What do you do when you come home from school? Do you go outside and play—or do you watch television or play a video game while you eat a snack?

Even thirty years ago, most children would have said they went outside and played after school, but these days, more

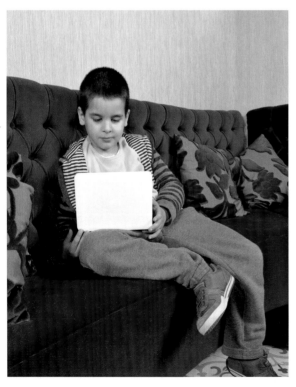

kids are watching television or sitting at the computer. There's nothing wrong with watching television or being on the computer, of course—you can learn a lot from both, especially if you watch the right shows and go to the best sites—but these activities have something in common: they're both done sitting down.

How much time do YOU spend watching television or playing on a computer?

So kids who have probably just spent most of their day sitting down at school, now come home and sit down again for the next few hours. Their parents are no different. Most adults work all day in jobs where they spend most of their time sitting, and then they too come home and watch television or sit at the computer some more.

In today's world, more and more people have a sit-down lifestyle. And that lifestyle is helping to build a big problem—more and more people are becoming **overweight** and **obese**.

What's the difference between being overweight and being obese? Both words mean that a person has too much body fat, so much so that it's a health risk. But a person who is obese has much more fat than a person who is overweight, and the health risks are greater as well.

A HEALTH PROBLEM

Lots of people think that being overweight is an appearance problem. In other words, they think people look better if they're thinner. But that's really not the point. People come in all different sizes and shapes—and no one should ever be insulted or treated with less respect because of their weight. People who are overweight or obese can still be smart and pretty and funny. But being overweight is actually a health problem.

Lots of health problems can come from being overweight or obese. If you weigh too much, the extra weight can damage your joints. It can change the way you breathe and sleep, and it can also change your moods, and energy levels. Your entire life can be changed by being overweight.

Children who are overweight or obese are more likely to get diabetes. This is a disease where your body doesn't break down sugar the way it should. If you have diabetes, you will probably have to take medicine or have special shots every day to help your body process sugar normally. Diabetes can lead to other diseases as well, including blindness. It can make it hard for you to heal after a cut or injury.

DID YOU KNOW?

Sometimes people think that those who are overweight are lazy or greedy. They think that if those people wanted to lose weight bad enough, they could easily become thinner. Sometimes people don't want to get to know others simply because they're overweight or obese. They assume that people with more fat are not as interesting, not as smart, or simply not as important.

Prejudice is the word we use when we think differently about others because of their race, their religion, or the way they look. Most of us know that this is wrong—but many people think it's okay to think about people differently because they are overweight or obese. This is a form of prejudice too. And yet we hear fat jokes at school all the time. Grownups tell fat jokes too. People on television do as well. Most of the time, people forget how mean this is, or how it makes others feel.

Being overweight also increases your chances of having heart disease. This is an illness we usually connect with older people, but carrying too much weight around is hard on your heart, no matter how old you are. Even worse, the heavier you are, the harder it will probably be for you to run around and exercise. Your heart and lungs need exercise to be healthy. Today, more and more children are obese or overweight—and more and more children are getting heart disease.

Overweight children are also likely to stay that way as they grow up. Being obese or overweight when you are an adult can put you at risk for even more diseases. Obesity may even cause certain kinds of **cancer**.

What is cancer? Cancer is a disease that causes the cells in different parts of your body to grow too fast, to the point that they kill healthy cells.

DID YOU KNOW?

A stereotype is a picture we have in our heads about a group of people. It's not necessarily true. In fact, it seldom is, because people are individuals, and each person within a group is different. But many people have a stereotype they use when they think about people who are overweight and obese. They may think people who are overweight are lazy, weak, and sad—or that they're not as clean or that they smell bad. Sometimes people think that those who are overweight and obese are not as smart and not as likeable as other people. And that's not true!

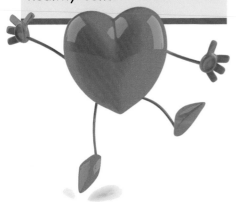

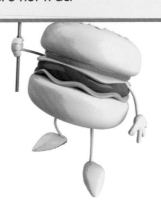

As people who are overweight or obese grow older, the added weight on their bodies can also lead to other problems, like **high blood pressure** (which increases your chances of having a **stroke**), **gallbladder** disease, and breathing problems. Being overweight can also mean that you have more problems handling your emotions. People who are obese or overweight are more likely to have **depression**.

What does high blood pressure and stroke mean? High blood pressure is when blood pushes against the walls of the blood vessels harder than is normal. This tends to happen when the vessels become too narrow. A stroke is when the cells in your brain suddenly die because they don't get enough blood.

What is your gallbladder? Your gallbladder is an organ in your body that helps you digest fats.

What is depression? Depression is an emotional illness that makes people feel very sad most of the time.

DID YOU KNOW?

Smoking is the number-one cause of deaths that could be prevented. Obesity is the number-two cause of all deaths that could otherwise have been prevented.

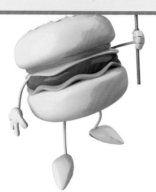

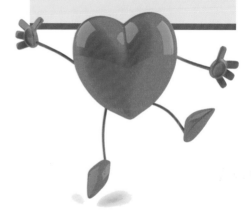

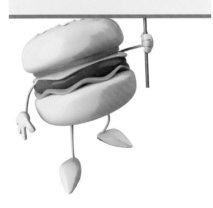

What is a tendency? If you have a tendency to do something, you are more likely to do it. Having a tendency to gain weight means you put on weight easily and have to work harder to stay at a healthy weight.

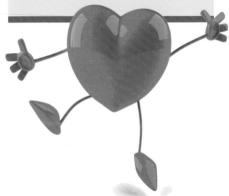

WHY DO PEOPLE BECOME OVERWEIGHT?

Obesity tends to run in families. In other words, your parents might pass on to you the **tendency** to gain weight more easily than other people do because you burn calories more slowly. During long-ago times, when food was often scarce, having a body that burned calories more slowly was a real advantage. But now that food is available all the time in most places in the world, this tendency works against you.

HOW DO YOU KNOW IF YOU'RE OVERWEIGHT?

Experts have figured out a way to help you know if you are in the healthy weight range for your height. It's called the body mass index or BMI.

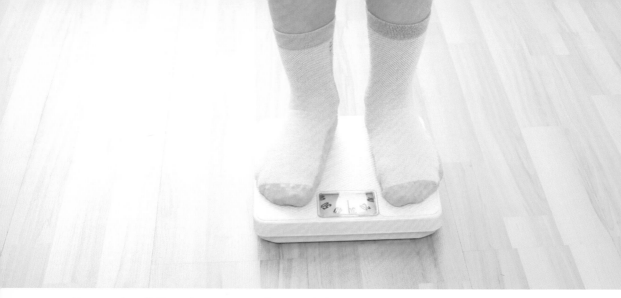

You can't tell if you're overweight simply by stepping on the scales.

The BMI formula uses height and weight to come up with a BMI number. Though the formula is the same for adults and children, figuring out what the BMI number means is a little more complicated for kids. For children, BMI is plotted on a growth chart that tells whether a child is underweight, healthy weight, overweight, or obese. Different BMI charts are used for boys and girls who are younger than twenty, because the amount of body fat differs between boys and girls. Also, the amount of body fat that is healthy is different, depending on whether you're a toddler or a teenager.

2 to 20 years: Boys
Body mass index-for-age percentiles

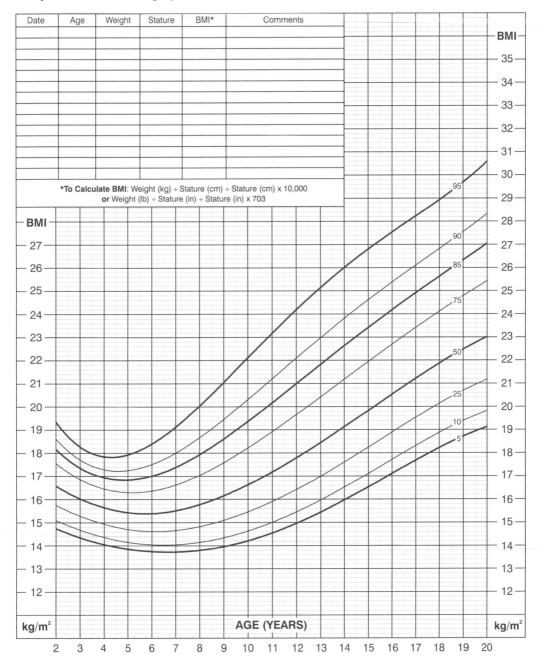

BMI growth chart for boys ages 2–20.

2 to 20 years: Girls
Body mass index-for-age percentiles

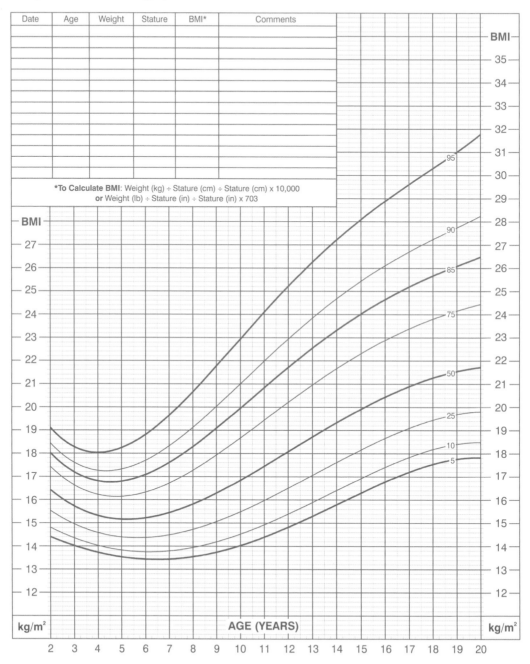

Date	Age	Weight	Stature	BMI*	Comments

*To Calculate BMI: Weight (kg) ÷ Stature (cm) ÷ Stature (cm) x 10,000
or Weight (lb) ÷ Stature (in) ÷ Stature (in) x 703

BMI growth chart for girls ages 2–20.

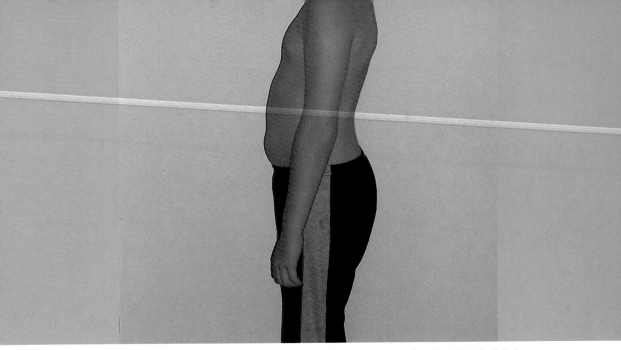

This boy is 5 feet and 1 inch tall, and he weighs 107 pounds. His BMI is 20.4, which means he is neither overweight nor underweight—he's in the normal weight range.

Each BMI chart is divided into percentiles. A child whose BMI is equal to or greater than the 5th percentile and less than the 85th percentile is considered a healthy weight for his or her age. A child at or above the 85th percentile but less than the 95th percentile for age is considered overweight. A child at or above the 95th percentile is considered obese. A child below the 5th percentile is considered underweight.

If you know how much you weigh and how tall you are, you can look at these charts and see for yourself whether you are overweight or obese—but it's also a good idea to talk to your doctor (even if that seems embarrassing). BMI is not always right, so a doctor will be better able to tell you if your weight is healthy or not.

Even though doctors use BMI to determine if you're overweight or obese, BMI is sometimes wrong. That's because different types of body tissues weigh different amounts. Muscle, for example, weighs eight or nine times as much as fat. This means that a small amount of muscle will be as heavy, or heavier, than a larger amount of fat.

Imagine two children who are the same height. One weighs 100 pounds. The other weighs 85 pounds. Judging by weight alone, you might think that the 85-pound child is healthier and has less fat than the 100-pound child. If the 100-pound kid, however, is very muscular, and the 85-pound kid has practically no muscles at all, then you'd be wrong. The 85-pound child could actually be both lighter and "fatter" than the muscular 100-pound kid.

A BIG PROBLEM

All around the world, more people are overweight today than ever before. This health problem affects young people as well as adults—one-third of all kids between the ages of two and nineteen are overweight or obese. That's a big problem for us all!

But it's also a complicated problem. Losing weight isn't easy, and there are no easy answers. Scientists agree, though: we're going to have to change the way we live. We need to move more!

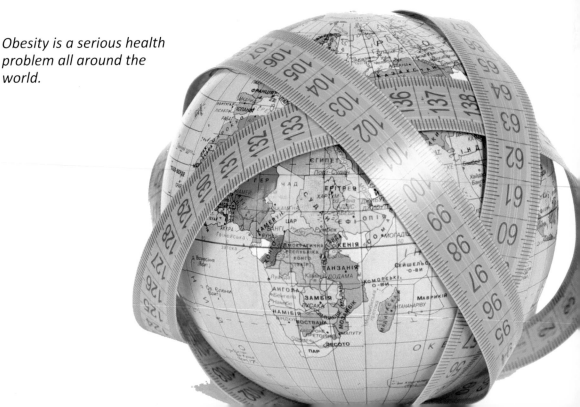

Obesity is a serious health problem all around the world.

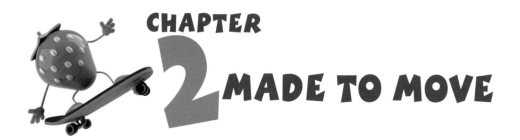

CHAPTER 2 MADE TO MOVE

Your body was made to move. Your muscles are designed to **expand** and **contract**, pulling your bones and bending your joints. Thousands of years ago, our ancestors spent their entire days walking, running, climbing, stretching, and throwing. Chasing animals for food, collecting food from plants, fighting off enemies: the effort it took just to survive kept people in great shape.

ENERGY

Moving your body takes energy —and your body gets **energy** from the food you eat. If your body was a car, your food would be the gasoline, the fuel your body burns to make it "run." All food gives you energy, but some foods give you more than others.

We talk about inches and feet (or centimeters and meters) when we want to

What does expand and contract mean? It means to get loose and then pull tight.

What is energy? Energy is the ability to be active, the power it takes to move.

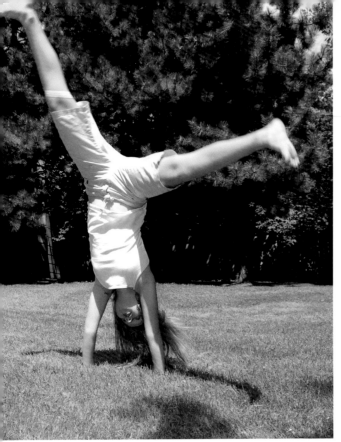

The more active you are, the more calories you'll burn during the day.

measure how long or tall something is; we use pints and quarts (or liters) to measure liquids like milk and soda—and we use calories to measure how much energy is in a certain food.

Each one of us needs a certain amount of calories every day to be healthy and have the energy we need for all the things we do in a day. Even sitting still takes a certain number of calories, but the more active we are, the more calories we need. A car that's sitting in the driveway doesn't need much fuel to keep it running—but a car that's driving fast out on the highway will need much more. Your body is the same.

DID YOU KNOW?

People who are bigger, more active, or who are growing usually need more calories than smaller people, people who don't move around very much, and people who aren't growing.

When we eat more calories than we need, our bodies store the extra energy as fat. Long ago, our ancestors went through times when they had plenty of food, followed by times when food was scarcer. Their bodies' stores of fat helped them get through the times when they had less food. Today, though, many times our bodies just keep storing more and more fat that never needs to be used. When that happens, we end up being overweight or obese.

Moving around is what your body is made to do. When you exercise regularly, you not only help your body use calories in a healthy way, you also make all the

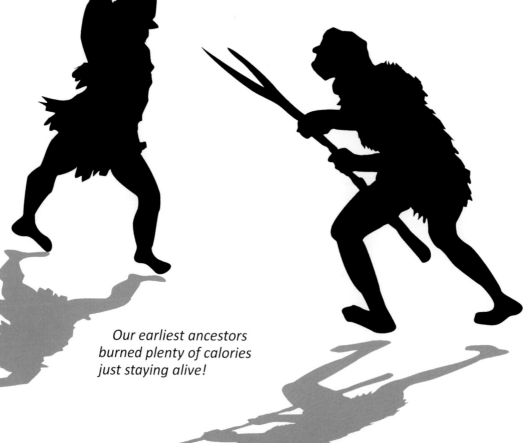

Our earliest ancestors burned plenty of calories just staying alive!

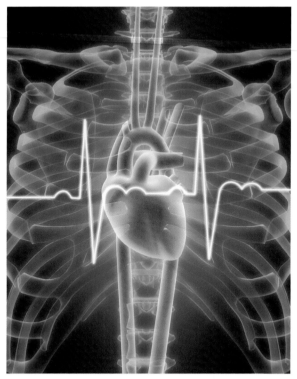
Your heart is made up of muscle.

cells and organs in your body healthier. When you're strong and fit, your body makes good use of the food you eat, and all your body parts are much more likely to work together the way they're supposed to. This means that even when you're not exercising, you burn more calories. You feel better, physically and emotionally—and you even think better!

EXERCISE AND YOUR HEART

You have big muscles in your arms and legs, and these get stronger when you exercise—but probably the most important muscle in your body is your heart. And it also gets stronger when you exercise.

Your heart works hard, pumping blood every day of your life. The blood carries oxygen to all the tiny cells in your body. The heart's job is what keeps you alive. Without oxygen, your cells would die. You would not be able to move or talk or think.

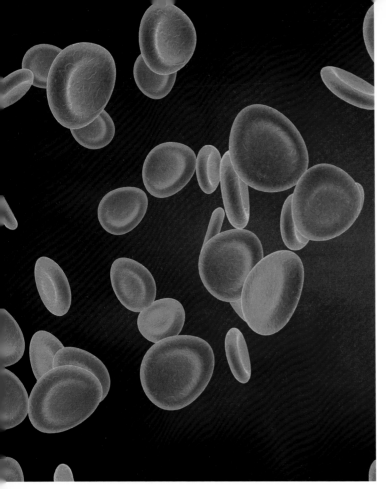

The red blood cells in your blood are what carry oxygen to all the cells of your body.

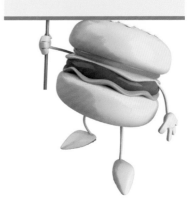

Your heart does this important job day after day, year after year, throughout your entire life. And when you exercise regularly, you help your heart do its job better—and odds are you will live longer.

The kind of exercise that is best for your heart is called aerobic exercise. "Aerobic" is a word that means "with air," and this kind of exercise means your body needs more oxygen than usual. You will breathe faster, and your heart will beat faster, pumping oxygen-carrying blood to all your cells. If you give your heart this kind of workout a few times every week, your heart will get even better at its job, delivering oxygen to all the parts of your body.

EXERCISE AND YOUR OTHER MUSCLES

Aerobic exercises are good for your heart, but another kind of exercise is better at making your muscles stronger. This kind of exercises doesn't make you breathe as fast when you're doing it, but it builds strength. By using your muscles to push or pull heavy weights, you can make them better able to do their job.

DID YOU KNOW?

These exercises and activities will help you build strong muscles:

push-ups
pull-ups
rowing
running
bike riding

Roller blading is good exercise!

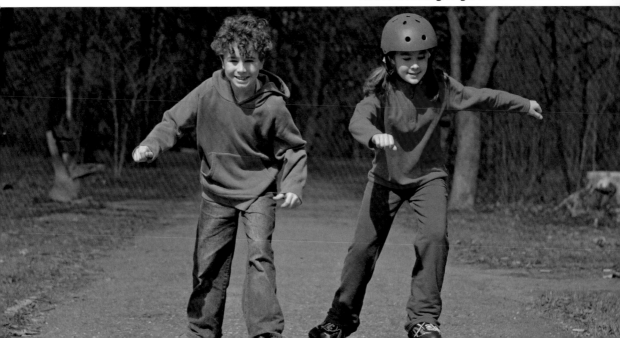

But you don't have to use a weight machine to do this kind of exercise. Your body is a weight, too, and when you lift it or move it, you are using strength. This kind of workout can make muscles bigger and stronger.

EXERCISE IS GOOD FOR YOUR BRAIN

You probably knew that exercise was good for your body. But did you know that exercise also helps you think better? Moving makes you breathe faster and your heart beat faster—and when you do, more blood flows to your brain. This means you can think more quickly and clearly.

Scientists have found that exercise actually improves our memories. Regular exercise helps you learn more easily and

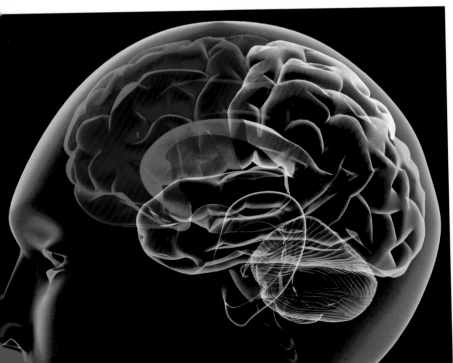

When you exercise, more blood gets to your brain—and that means you can think better.

think things through faster. It helps you concentrate. So if you want to be a better student, exercise!

EXERCISE MAKES YOU FEEL GOOD

It feels good to have a strong body that is able to have fun playing games and sports. But you don't have to be an athlete to enjoy exercise. Everyone feels better with a body that's strong and healthy.

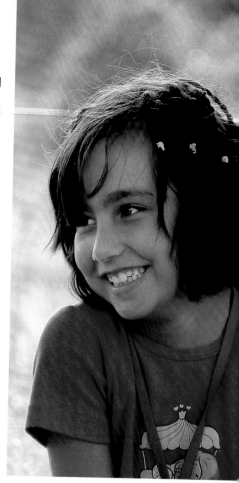

Exercise also makes you feel happier because it causes your body to send chemicals called endorphins into your bloodstream. These chemicals improve your mood.

Exercise makes you feel happier!

If you exercise regularly, you're less likely to feel sad and discouraged for very long. Life can be hard sometimes, and everyone gets upset—but exercise helps you cope with life's challenges. It releases some of the stress and tension that everyone feels sometimes.

So if exercise is so great, why don't we do it more? Well, mostly, because there are only so many hours in the day—and we spend those hours doing other things.

CHAPTER 3
NOT ENOUGH EXERCISE

Every day, there are certain things you have to do. When you're a kid, going to school is one of those things. As an adult, you'll probably have to go to work instead. That's just the way things are, and hopefully, you enjoy school most of the time, and one day you'll have a job you enjoy as well. But there's no getting around the fact that school and work take up a lot of the day. Most kids spend about seven or eight hours in school, and most of the hours are probably spent sitting at a desk.

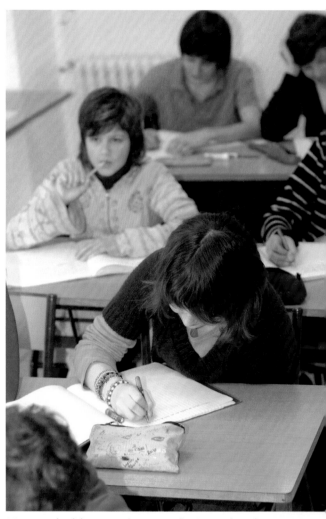

You probably spend most of your school day sitting at a desk.

Since each day has twenty-four hours in it, that leaves you about sixteen hours. But if you're a kid, you need to spend at least ten of those hours sleeping. So now you're down to six hours. During those hours, you have to eat and go to the bathroom and do your homework and talk to your family and friends. Say that takes a couple of hours. Now you're left with four hours.

So far, none of the things you've done during your day have involved much moving around. If you're going to exercise, you're going to need to do it in those four hours.

But most kids don't.

A CHANGING WORLD

A hundred years ago, even fifty years ago, most grownups

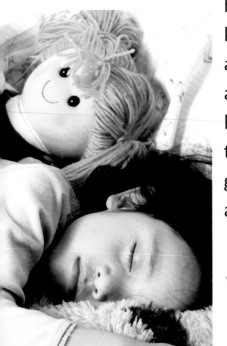

had plenty of physical work to do that kept them active. Keeping a house clean and growing food took up a lot of time—and burned a lot of calories. Children had chores to do, as well, and when their chores were done, children played games like tag and hide-and-go-seek and hopscotch. All these games involved

You need to sleep at least ten hours every night.

MOVING. In those days, people moved their bodies every single day.

But that's not the way we live today. Labor-saving inventions like washing machines and vacuum cleaners mean we can keep our homes and clothing clean without working so hard. We buy our food at the grocery store, and often, our food comes in quick, easy-to-fix packages—or we eat out at a restaurant. Daily life just doesn't take as much effort as it once did.

DID YOU KNOW?

Scientists are studying families to better understand what's making kids overweight. They found that families' habits have a big part in whether kids gain weight. The children who are least likely to be obese or overweight eat dinner with their families six or seven times a week, sleep for at least 10.5 hours each night, and watch less than two hours of television per day.

A hundred years ago, children your age spent most of their free time playing active games like crack-the-whip or tag.

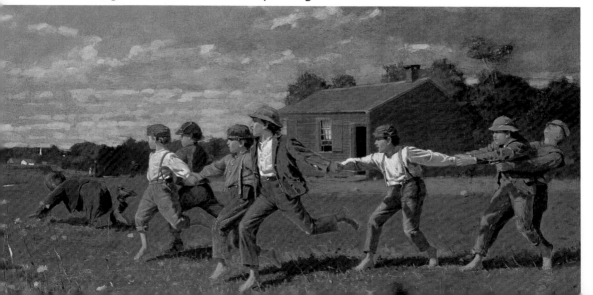

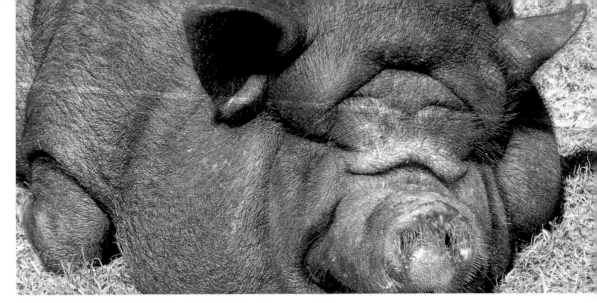

Animals who don't move around much also get fat.

That seems like a good thing. After all, if we have less work to do, then we have more time to enjoy ourselves. And that would be fine—except the things we do today to enjoy ourselves often don't involve moving our bodies.

Scientists did an experiment with rats and pigs, where they kept the animals still and didn't let them run around. Then the scientists tested the animals to find out what was going on inside their bodies. The scientists discovered that the animals that didn't run around for hours no longer had very much of a chemical called lipase in their bodies. Lipase helps break down fat molecules. Without so much lipase in their bodies, the animals stopped burning calories as fuel—and started getting fat instead.

So the **researchers** decided next to find out what happens to human beings who sit still for long periods of time. They found that not moving around for hours in a row does the same thing to people that it does to rats and pigs—it makes them stop burning calories and start getting fat.

What are researchers?
They're people who do experiments and try to find the answers to questions.

IT'S NOT YOUR FAULT!

If you're a kid, you didn't choose your family's lifestyle. You certainly didn't choose the way the entire world lives around you. You were just born into this world, a world where people don't move as much as they should. So don't blame yourself if you don't move enough to keep your body healthy.

But you CAN do something about it!

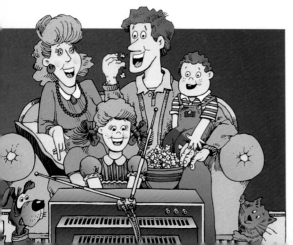

The invention of the television changed the way most families live their lives. Sitting down to watch a TV show in the evening (often while snacking) now became a way of life.

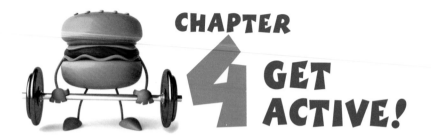

CHAPTER 4 GET ACTIVE!

Maybe you like sports. If you do, sports are a great way to get the exercise you need to be healthy. Play as much basketball, softball, soccer, hockey, lacrosse, or tennis as you can.

Sometimes, though, kids don't like organized sports because they were once on a team and they didn't have fun. If you try a sport, and all the other kids seem to know what they're doing while you don't, you can feel shy and embarrassed. Or maybe you don't like the pressure of competing against other teams,

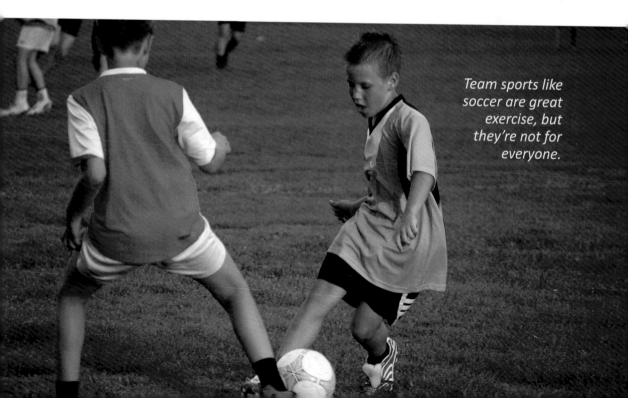

Team sports like soccer are great exercise, but they're not for everyone.

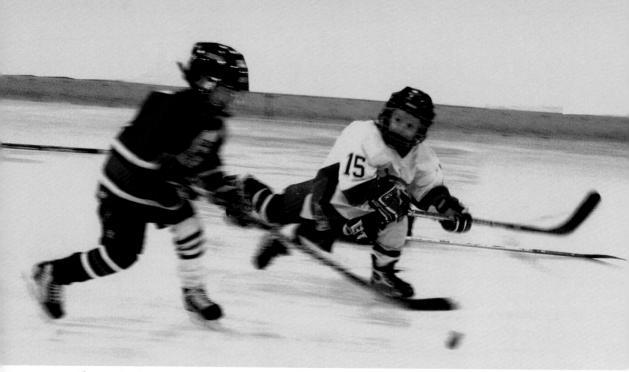

If you don't enjoy one team sport, don't assume you won't like a different one. Try a few!

where you know one team is going to win and the other is going to lose. Competition can make some kids get so excited about winning that they get angry and yell at a player who makes a mistake. If you were the player who made the mistake, it can make you feel like crawling under a rock!

If that's happened to you, don't give up. Almost everyone has had this happen, because EVERYBODY makes mistakes sometimes. If you've had a bad experience with a team, try a new sport or a new league. Some programs emphasize skill building over competition, and some leagues don't even keep score. Being on a team can be a lot of fun, and it's a great way to get the exercise your body needs.

There are dozens of sports, so you might not have found the right one for you yet. Different sports require different skills, so if you try a few sports, you'll be more likely to find one that suits you. And if you don't like being on a team that much, you might like individual sports better. An individual sport means you do the sport on your own or with just one or two other people, instead of on a team. You can do these sports competitively or just for the fun of doing them. Here's a list of some individual sports:

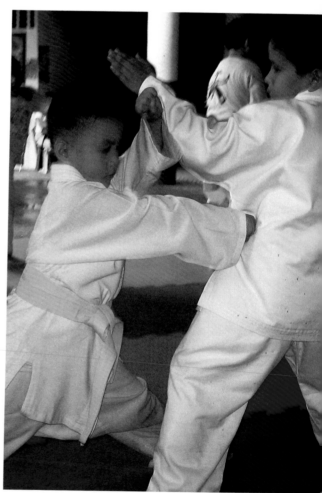

- swimming
- running
- wrestling
- tennis
- skateboarding
- in-line skating
- biking
- martial arts
- bowling

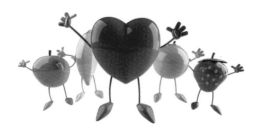

The martial arts are a great way to get exercise.

But being active isn't really about sports. Sports can be a lot of fun, and they're a good way to get exercise. But you don't have to become an athlete or even take part in any sport at all. You can still change your lifestyle and move more.

OTHER WAYS TO BE ACTIVE

There are lots of other ways to have fun moving your body. Here are just a few ideas:

- playing at a playground
- playing with your dog
- raking leaves
- jumping rope
- washing the car
- playing hide-and-seek
- hiking
- playing tag
- dancing
- cleaning the house
- playing with a Frisbee

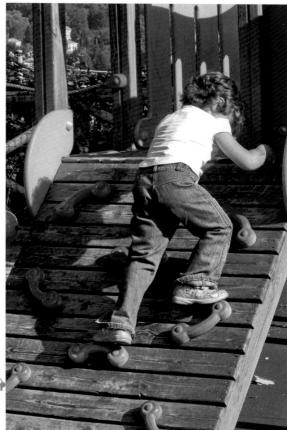

A playground is a fun place to get the exercise your body needs.

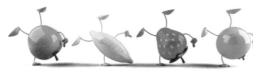

Exercise should be fun. So pick something you genuinely enjoy doing. You'll be more likely to make exercise a habit if you like what you're doing.

MAKING AN EXERCISE PLAN

Here are some suggestions that might help you make exercise a habit:

• Talk to your parents first. Explain why exercise is so important, and get their permission for whatever forms of exercise you choose to do. If you'll need rides or if your exercise schedule is going to cut into your parents' lives in some way, make sure you have their support.

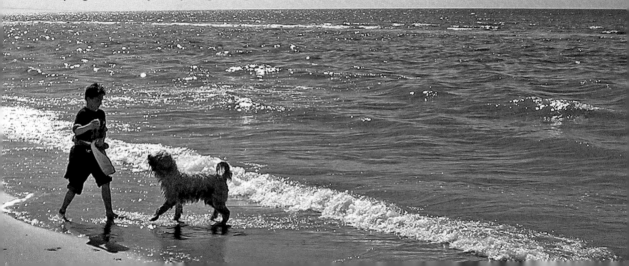

Playing with the family dog is a good way to get exercise too.

- Encourage your family to exercise with you. Maybe your family could get a membership at a health club or the YMCA. Choose more active outings for family days together—hiking instead of going to a movie, for example, or swimming instead of staying home and watching television.

- Use the buddy system. If you have a friend who will exercise with you, you'll have more fun, and you'll be more likely to stick with it.

- Keep an exercise diary. Write down the days you exercise, the distance or length of time of your workout, and how you feel after each session.

Find active things your family enjoys doing together, like swimming on a hot day.

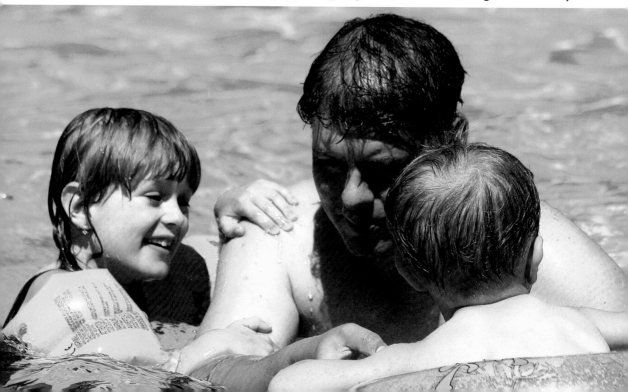

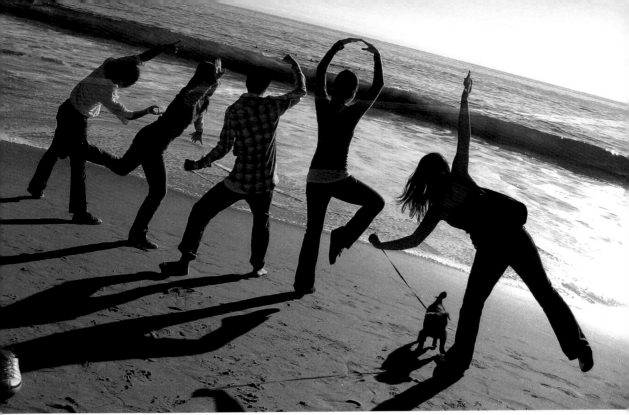

Exercise is more fun if you do it with friends!

- Don't push yourself too hard. You should be able to talk while you're exercising. If you can't, because you're breathing too hard, then you need to slow down your pace a little. Build your strength gradually.
- If you miss a day, plan a make-up day. Don't double your exercise time during your next session. If you do, you're more likely to get too tired—if you're too tired, exercising won't seem like as much fun—and if you don't think exercise is fun, you're not as likely to keep doing it!
- If your form of exercise needs good weather, have a back-up indoor exercise plan for rainy days.

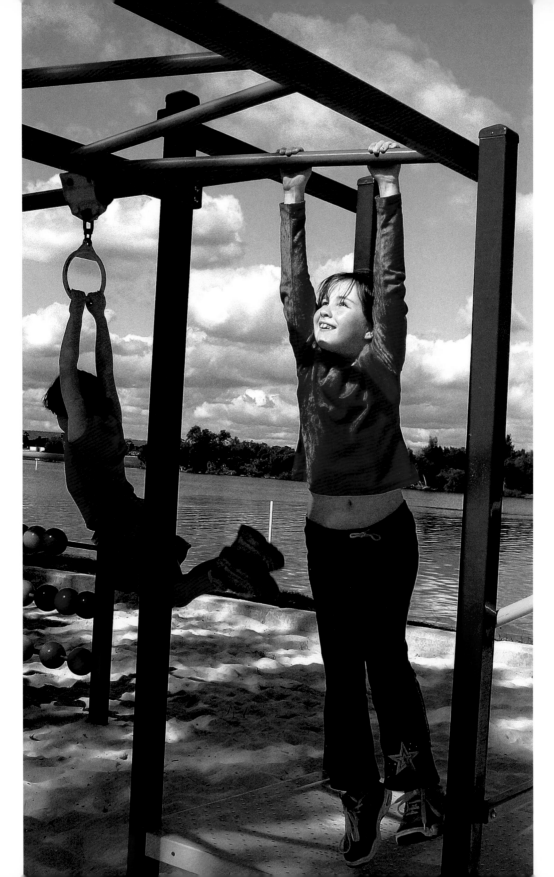

- Try something new. Take lessons to learn a new sport.
- Do different things different days, so you won't get bored. Take a walk one day, for example, go swimming the next, and then go for a bike ride on the weekend
- Try not to compare yourself with others. Having a strong healthy body doesn't mean you have to be a skilled athlete or win prizes. Being physically fit is about being in the best shape possible for YOU, regardless of how that compares with others.
- Be ready to change your exercise plan when needed. Any time there's a change in your family's routine, that will probably mean you have to build exercise back into your life all over again. For instance, if your mom starts a new job, she may not be able to pick you up anymore after basketball practice. Or when school lets out for the summer, you may finder it harder to keep up with your exercise program, even though you

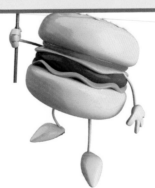

DID YOU KNOW?

The National Association for Sports and Physical Education recommends that school-age kids:

- get 1 hour or more of physical activity on most or all days.
- also take part in several periods of physical activity of 15 minutes or more each day.
- avoid sitting still for 2 hours or more.

Try to have at least an hour of active play every day.

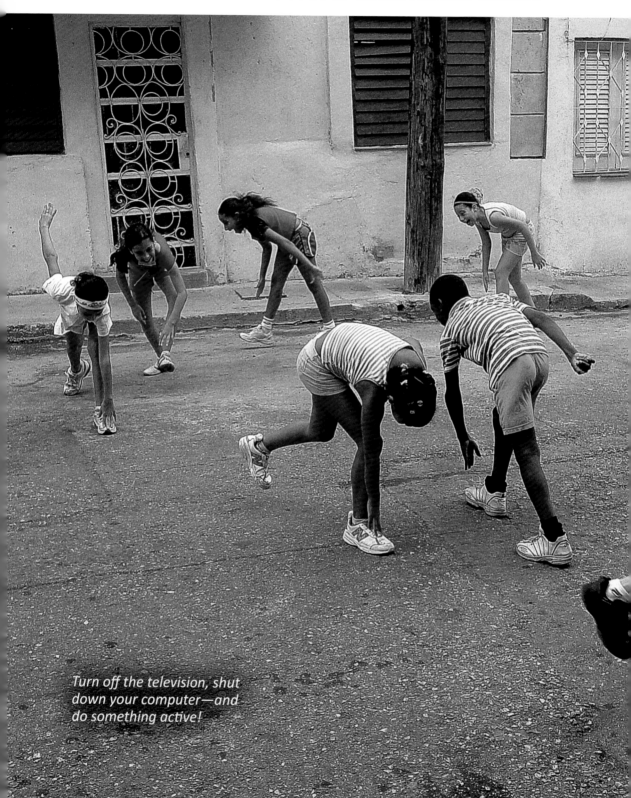

Turn off the television, shut down your computer—and do something active!

have more time. That's only normal. It just means you have to find new ways to build exercise back into your life again.

- Don't give up! Sometimes you won't feel like exercising and you'll just flop down and watch some TV instead. Don't feel angry with yourself—and don't get discouraged and drop your exercise plan altogether. Just get yourself going the next time. The more you exercise, the easier it will get—and the more it will become a habit for you.

So turn off the television, let your computer go to sleep, and think of something else to do every day, something that will move your body and burn calories. Remember, it really doesn't matter HOW you move—so long as you move!

READ MORE ABOUT IT

Bean, Anita. *Awesome Foods for Active Kids: The ABCs of Eating for Energy and Health*. Alameda, Calif.: Hunter House, 2006.

Behan, Eileen. *Fit Kids: Raising Physically and Emotionally Strong Kids with Real Food.* New York: Pocket Publishing, 2001.

Berg, Frances M. *Children and Teens Afraid to Eat*. Hettinger, N.D.: Healthy Weight Network, 2001.

Dolgoff, Joanna. *Red Light, Green Light, Eat Right: The Food Solution That Lets Kids Be Kids.* Emmaus, Penn.: Rodale, 2009.

Gaesser, Glenn. *Big Fat Lies: The Truth About Your Weight and Your Health.* Carlsbad, Calif.: Gürze Books, 2002.

Johnson, Susan and Laurel Mellin. *Just for Kids!* (Obesity Prevention Workbook). San Anselmo, Calif.: Balboa Publishing, 2002.

Lillien, Lisa. *Hungry Girl 1-2-3: The Easiest, Most Delicious, Guilt-Free Recipes on the Planet*. New York: St. Martin's, 2010.

Vos, Miriam B. *The No-Diet Obesity Solution for Kids.* Bethesda, Md.: AGA Institute, 2009.

Wann, Marilyn. *Fat! So? Because You Don't Have to Apologize for Your Size.* Berkeley. Calif.: Ten Speed Press, 2009.

Zinczenko, David and Matt Goulding. *Eat This Not That! For Kids!* Emmaus, Penn.: Rodale, 2008.

FIND OUT MORE ON THE INTERNET

About Our Kids: Obesity and Overweight
www.aboutourkids.org/aboutour/articles/gr_obesity_03.html

Activity Cards
www.bam.gov/sub_physicalactivity/physicalactivity_activitycards.html

Aim for a Healthy Weight: Assess Your Risk
www.nhlbi.nih.gov/health/public/heart/obesity/lose_wt/risk.htm#limitations

American Obesity Association
www.obesity.org

Environmental Contributions to Obesity
www.endotext.org/obesity/obesity7/obesity7.htm

The Learning Center
www.hebs.scot.nhs.uk/learningcentre/obesity/intro/index.cfm

Obesity: Causes
www.weight-loss-i.com/obesity-causes.htm

Obesity and Environment Factsheet
www.niehs.nih.gov/oc/factsheets/obesity.htm

Move It!
www.fns.usda.gov/tn/tnrockyrun/moveit.htm

MyPyramid Blast Off Game
www.mypyramid.gov/kids/kids_game.html

Small Step Kids
www.smallstep.gov/kids/html/games_and_activities.html

The websites listed on this page were active at the time of publication. The publisher is not responsible for websites that have changed their address or discontinued operation since the date of publication. The publisher will review and update the websites upon each reprint.

INDEX

PICTURE CREDITS

ABOUT THE AUTHOR

Rae Simons has ghostwritten several adult books on dieting and obesity. She is also the author of more than thirty young adult books. She lives in upstate New York, where she tries hard to get enough exercise and eat healthy foods.

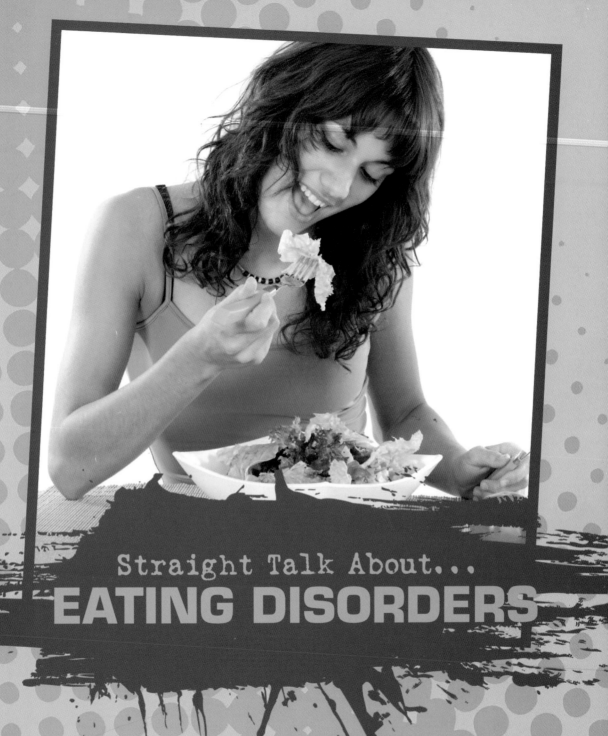

Straight Talk About...
EATING DISORDERS

Carrie Iorizzo

Crabtree Publishing Company
www.crabtreebooks.com

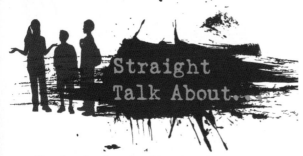

Straight
Talk About...

Developed and produced by: Netscribes Inc.

Author: Carrie Iorizzo

Publishing plan research and development:
Sean Charlebois, Reagan Miller
Crabtree Publishing Company

Project Controller: Sandeep Kumar G

Editorial director: Kathy Middleton

Editors: John Perritano, Molly Aloian

Proofreader: Kathy Middleton

Art director: Dibakar Acharjee

Designer: Shruti Aggarwal

Cover design: Margaret Amy Salter

Production coordinator and
prepress technician: Margaret Amy Salter

Print coordinators: Katherine Berti,
Margaret Amy Salter

Consultant: Carla Lundblade, M.S., L.P.C., N.C.C.

Photographs:
Cover: Jaimie Duplass/Shutterstock; Title Page: Gelpi
JM/Shutterstock Inc.; p.4: Piotr Marcinski/Shutterstock
Inc.; p.6: Kekyalyaynen/Shutterstock Inc.; p.8: Monkey
Business Images/Shutterstock Inc.; p.9: Mark Herreid /
Shutterstock Inc.; p.10: Catalin Petolea/ Shutterstock
Inc.; p.13: Yuri Arcurs/Shutterstock Inc.; p.14: Monkey
Business Images/Shutterstock Inc.; p.15: NotarYES/
Shutterstock Inc.; p.16: Elena Elisseeva/Shutterstock
Inc.; p.19: Shutterstock Inc.; p.20: Stuart Monk/
Shutterstock Inc.; p.22: Orhan Cam/Shutterstock Inc.;
p.24: Piotr Marcinski/Shutterstock Inc.; p.25: PHOTO
FUN/Shutterstock Inc.; p.26: Sergey Peterman/
Shutterstock Inc.; p.28: Daniel_Dash/Shutterstock Inc.;
p.31: Ariwasabi/Shutterstock Inc.; p.32: Martin
Allinger/Shutterstock Inc.; p.34: OLJ Studio/
Shutterstock Inc.; p.35: Kolobrod/Shutterstock Inc.;
p.36: REATISTA/Shutterstock Inc.; p.38.1: Sweet
November studio/Shutterstock Inc.; p.38.2: TrotzOlga/
Shutterstock Inc.; p.40: pedalist/Shutterstock Inc.;
p.42:wrangler/Shutterstock Inc.

Library and Archives Canada Cataloguing in Publication

Iorizzo, Carrie
    Eating disorders / Carrie Iorizzo.

(Straight talk about--)
Includes index.
Issued also in electronic format.
ISBN 978-0-7787-2183-3 (bound).--ISBN 978-0-7787-2190-1 (pbk.)

    1. Eating disorders--Juvenile literature. I. Title. II. Series:
Straight talk about-- (St. Catharines, Ont.)

RC552.E18I67 2013   j616.85'26   C2013-900981-7

Library of Congress Cataloging-in-Publication Data

Iorizzo, Carrie.
    Eating disorders / Carrie Iorizzo.
        pages cm -- (Straight talk about)
    Includes index.
    ISBN 978-0-7787-2183-3 (reinforced library binding) --
ISBN 978-0-7787-2190-1 (pbk.) -- ISBN 978-1-4271-9066-6
(electronic pdf) -- ISBN 978-1-4271-9120-5 (electronic html)
    1. Eating disorders--Juvenile literature. 2. Eating disorders in
adolescence--Juvenile literature. 3. Self-perception--Juvenile
literature. I. Title.

RC552.E18I587 2013
616.85'26--dc23
                                        2013004642

Crabtree Publishing Company

www.crabtreebooks.com   1-800-387-7650

Printed in the USA/052013/JA20130412

Published in Canada
Crabtree Publishing
616 Welland Ave.
St. Catharines, ON
L2M 5V6

Published in the United States
Crabtree Publishing
PMB 59051
350 Fifth Avenue, 59th Floor
New York, New York 10118

Published in the United Kingdom
Crabtree Publishing
Maritime House
Basin Road North, Hove
BN41 1WR

Published in Australia
Crabtree Publishing
3 Charles Street
Coburg North
VIC, 3058

CONTENTS

Nicki stood naked in front of the full-length mirror in the bathroom. No matter how many times she threw up, she just couldn't get rid of that fat blob on her hips.

Nicki stepped on the scale and watched the red needle hover over the 95-pound mark. *Ninety-five pounds—I'm such a fat slob! I'm pathetic. I ate three pieces of chocolate cake, a bag of barbecue chips, and all the leftover potato salad.*

Nicki rifled through a drawer until she found the *Ipecac*. Without measuring, she tipped her head back and drained the dark liquid from the bottle.

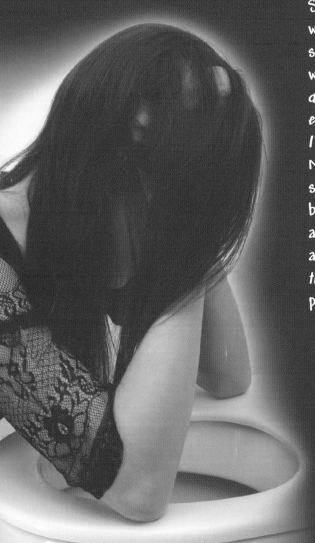

She sat on the toilet seat and waited. Soon, the Ipecac would start to work, and all that food would be down the toilet. *Never again,* she promised. *I'll never eat again. But mom was right. I'm a pig when it comes to food.* Nicki braced herself as her stomach began to churn. She began to vomit. Her throat was always sore from puking, almost as sore as her stomach. *This time would be different,* she promised. *No more food.*

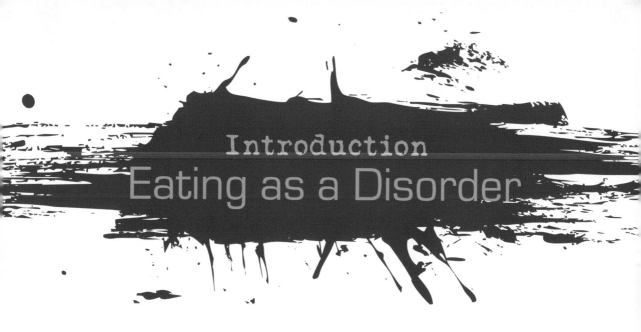

Nicki, like millions of others, has an eating disorder. An eating disorder is a type of mental illness. Eating disorders are complicated. Scientists and researchers have identified some of the factors that play a role in eating disorders, also known as ED. Some of those factors include: family environment, cultural background, *genes*, peer pressure, and stress.

There are three main types of eating disorders: anorexia nervosa, bulimia nervosa, and compulsive-eating disorder. Other eating disorders that are not as well known include purging disorder, night-eating syndrome, and orthorexia, in which a person obsesses about eating healthy foods.

When most people think about eating disorders they think of girls like Nicki. But eating disorders affect both girls and boys. Some studies say boys are good at hiding an eating disorder. It's estimated that there are more than a million adolescent boys in the United States who suffer from eating disorders.

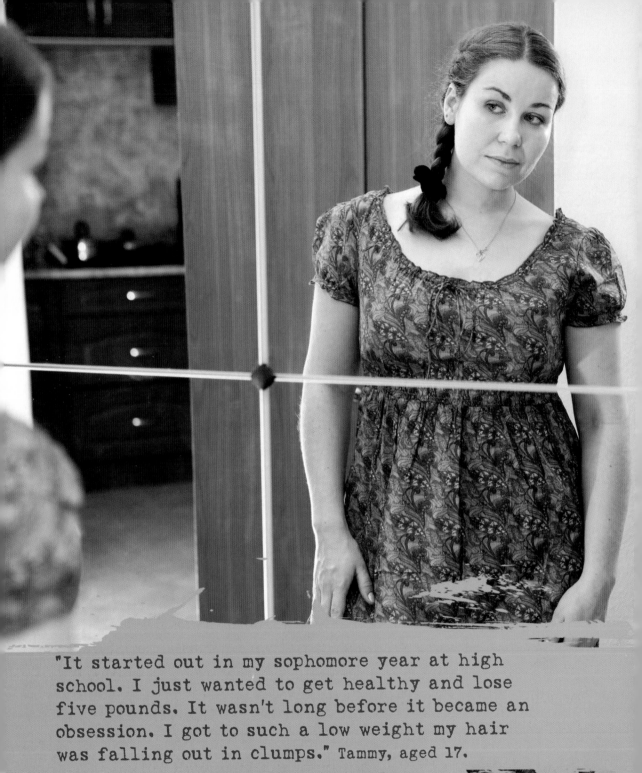

"It started out in my sophomore year at high school. I just wanted to get healthy and lose five pounds. It wasn't long before it became an obsession. I got to such a low weight my hair was falling out in clumps." Tammy, aged 17.

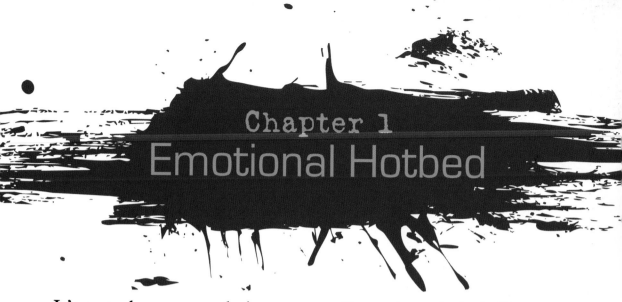

Chapter 1
Emotional Hotbed

It's not always easy being young. Sometimes it feels like no one is listening. Nothing you wear looks good. Your biceps just won't pop. No one understands.

Such feelings are normal. If these feelings become extreme, they might affect your daily routine and cause stress and poor health. Self-critical thoughts, negative feelings about body image, food, and weight gain, might be the beginnings of an eating disorder.

ED can start out innocently. You might want to drop five pounds to fit into a new bathing suit or just want to eat healthier and work on those abdominal muscles. These are all great ideas, but when mixed with a fatal dash of poor self-esteem, identity issues, and problems at home or school, you may find yourself developing a serious health issue.

Food becomes a crutch that helps you deal with larger issues that are often too hard to face, too painful to deal with, or just too embarrassing.

Big Problem

Eating disorders in the United States affect two kids out of every 100, including boys. In Canada, 37 percent of Grade 9 girls and 40 percent of Grade 10 girls think they're too fat. Twenty-five percent of adolescent boys get teased about their weight at school and at home. In 2002, 1.5 percent of all Canadian women between the ages of 15 and 24 had an eating disorder.

Eating can be fun, but eating disorders are a problem both males and females face each day.

By the Numbers

- In the United States, almost 24 million people have an eating disorder.
- One study estimates that 0.9 percent of females and 0.3 percent of all males that have anorexia nervosa will have it their entire lives. Of those who suffer from bulimia nervosa, 1.5 percent of females and 0.5 percent of males will deal with it their entire lives.
- In Canada, about 10 to 20 percent of people with eating disorders die from medical problems.

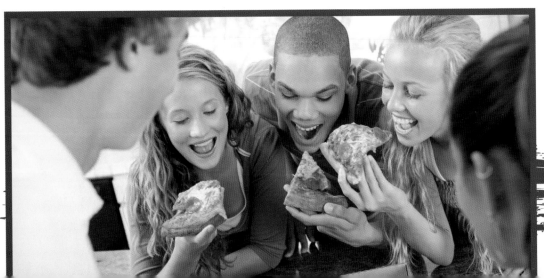

What's Healthy?

What does it mean to be healthy? First, being healthy means eating when you're hungry and making smart food choices every day.

Being healthy also means exercising for one hour a day, but not overdoing it. It means eating five servings—about 2.5 cups (600 mL)—of fruits and vegetables each day. It means choosing whole grains and lean proteins. It involves avoiding fast foods, fatty foods, and sugary foods and drinks.

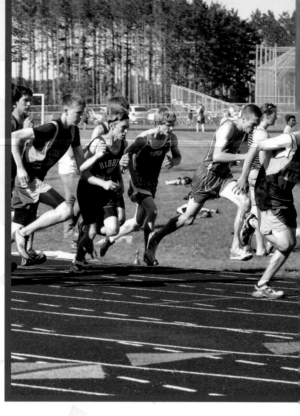

Maintaining a nutritious diet coupled with moderate exercise contributes to healthy weight management.

It also means treating yourself on occasion. Eating a piece of chocolate cake now and then can make just about any day perfect.

The American Heart Association recommends that girls between the ages of 9 and 13 consume 1,600 **calories** a day. Girls between the ages of 14 to 18 should eat 1,800 calories a day. For boys between 9 and 13, the suggested calorie amount is 1,800. For those between the ages of 14 to 18, it's 2,200 calories per day.

If you're on a sports team or on the go all the time, you should eat a little more.

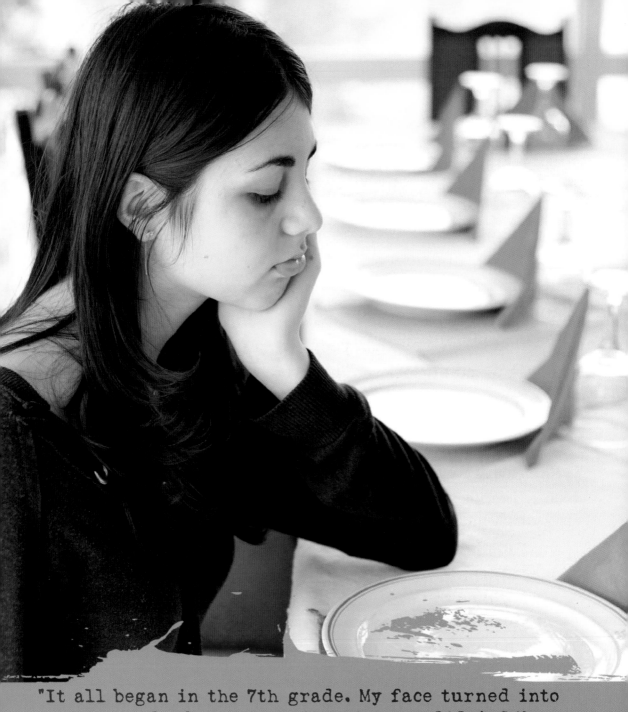

"It all began in the 7th grade. My face turned into a pizza, and I began to gain weight. I didn't like myself, or anyone else, for that matter. I became depressed and suicidal. I was just the "fat girl."
Jami, aged 15.

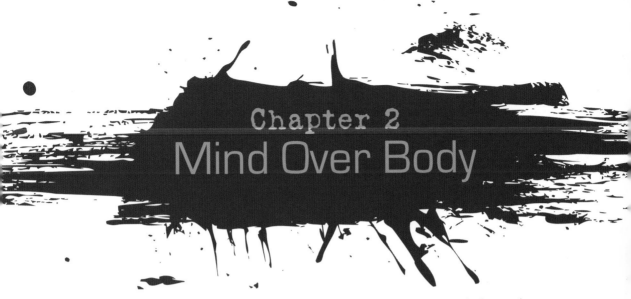

Chapter 2
Mind Over Body

A mental illness is a medical condition involving the mind. Decades ago, people with mental illnesses were shunned by society. They were often locked away in special institutions where they received little treatment. Today, we understand that good mental health is just as important as being in good physical health. Having a mental illness means you have a treatable condition.

ED, like any other mental illness, can change the way you think, how you act, and how you behave. Having an eating disorder can sometimes make it difficult to cope with simple things, such as getting up in the morning, going to school, hanging with your friends, or helping around the house. It can also affect your mood and how you feel about yourself. Having ED is nothing to be ashamed of, though. With help, it can be treated.

Danger Zone

Age and gender are two of the main risk factors when it comes to developing ED. Preteens, teens, and young adults are more at risk of developing eating disorders than older people. However, eating disorders are becoming common in younger children and older adults. Moreover, females are more at risk than males. The University of Maryland Medical Center estimates that 7 million females and 1 million males in the United States have an eating disorders.

Another risk factor is **ethnicity**. Although eating disorders occur in every race and culture, Caucasian, or white, females tend to have the highest risk.

Why is that? Television, movies, magazines, the Internet, advertising, and peer pressure all combine to make young people sensitive about their body images. The constant images of attractive models and thin movie stars can make most of us feel self-conscious about the shape of our bodies.

By the Numbers

- Almost 50 percent of people with eating disorders suffer from depression.
- Only 1 out of 10 people with an eating disorder seeks therapy.
- In the United States, almost 24 million people have some form of eating disorder.
- Eating disorders are the cause of more deaths than any other mental illness.

Source: National Association of Anorexia Nervosa and Associated Disorders

More Factors

Certain personality traits, including low self-esteem, the fear of losing control, inappropriate self-discipline, dependency, and the inability to interact with others, can be contributing factors to ED. Some mental illnesses, such as anxiety disorders, depression, and **oppositional defiant disorder**, a condition in which a person is aggressive to anyone in authority, are also associated with eating disorders.

A person might also be **genetically predisposed** to an eating disorder. Researchers have found that if one identical twin has an eating disorder, the other twin will likely suffer from it, too. They also found that people with relatives who have anorexia are eight times more likely to develop the condition than a person who does not have a relative with ED. Scientists have also linked a specific **chromosome**, called chromosome 10, to bulimia and **obesity**. A certain protein in the brain may also put some people at risk.

Although there is no one cause for ED, a preoccupation with your body and weight is high on the list. Many other causes are related to family influences.

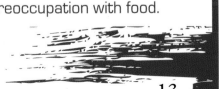

Obsession with body shape is common in most eating disorders, as is intense fear of gaining weight and preoccupation with food.

13

All in the Family

Studies have found that girls between the ages of 9 and 10 usually go on diets at the insistence of their mothers. If mom had, or has, an eating disorder, her daughter or daughters will probably have an eating disorder, too. Sexual abuse by family members can also trigger eating disorders in females. Researchers have also found that young boys are heavily influenced by their fathers' disapproval of their weight.

Children whose parents abuse drugs and alcohol often use food as a way to feel in control of their lives. Some teens might suffer from eating disorders if obesity runs in the family.

While the environment in which a person lives plays a role in developing an eating disorder, medical problems are also to blame. Abnormalities in the brain's hypothalamus, which controls behavior, or the amygdala, which plays a role in depression and anxiety, often contribute to the onset of eating disorders. Moreover, hormones that affect stress, appetite, hunger, and metabolism, have an effect.

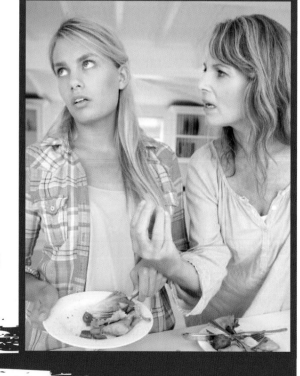

Family environment is often a good indication of whether you will be stricken with an eating disorder.

Warning Signs

Sometimes it's hard to know if a person has an eating disorder. Each has specific symptoms, but here are some general signs to look for:

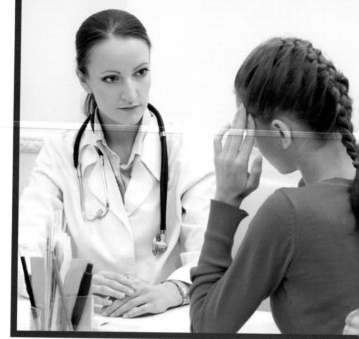

Getting help is important for anyone suffering from an eating disorder.

- looking too thin
- tired all the time
- wearing baggy clothes that do not fit properly
- always making excuses to avoid meals and eating
- constant preoccupation with food
- extremely afraid of gaining weight
- concerned about body shape
- avoiding friends and fun activities
- obsessed with exercising
- hiding food
- throwing away uneaten meals
- tiredness, dizziness, and fainting
- vomiting after eating
- swollen jawline, bloodshot eyes, calluses on the knuckles—all indications of vomiting
- always cold, even when it's warm
- irregular, or absent, monthly **menstrual** periods
- moody, withdrawn, secretive, irritable, or depressed

15

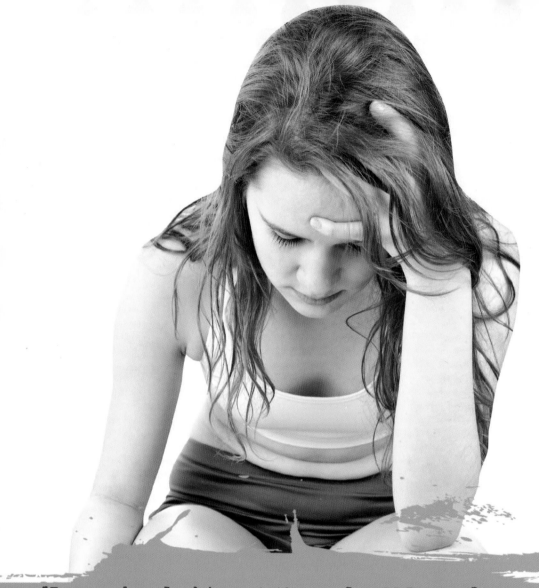

"I remember looking at the scale--115 pounds, and I wanted to be 100 pounds. I ate nothing and started drinking water and exercising too much. One day, when I was running cross country, I passed out. An ambulance took me to the hospital. Doctors said I had anorexia." Anonymous, aged 16.

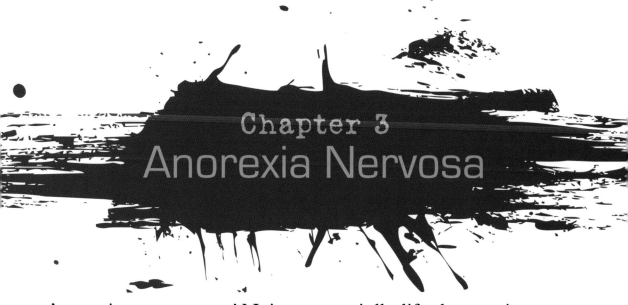

Chapter 3
Anorexia Nervosa

Anorexia nervosa, or AN, is a potentially life-threatening mental illness. It is categorized by severe weight loss caused by self-starvation. People with AN are frightened about gaining weight. They will go to great lengths to maintain a body weight much lower than what is healthy for their age and height.

People suffering from AN not only have the intense fear of gaining weight, but they have distorted perceptions of their bodies. They often deny that they are hungry. Still, anorexic people remain preoccupied with food and often cook for themselves and others.

AN affects both males and females, although more girls than boys suffer from the disorder.

The Perfect Body?

Although anorexia centers on food, its roots go much deeper as a person tries to gain control and to achieve the so-called "perfect body." They regulate their food intake by using **laxatives,** and **diuretics,** or by exercising excessively.

There are two subtypes of anorexia. Restricting anorexia is the classic form of the condition, in which people maintain a low body weight by carefully regulating the foods they eat. They might constantly exercise or starve themselves to bring their weight down.

Binging (and **purging**) is another type of anorexia. A binger will eat large quantities of food and then purge, or force themselves, to vomit.

White females are more likely to suffer from anorexia than any other group. About 10 percent of young males will also develop anorexia.

Eating disorders, such as anorexia, tend to run in families, especially those that are goal-oriented. How do you know if you or someone you love has anorexia? Some of the risk factors include:

- being worried about your weight and body shape
- having anxiety as a child
- having eating problems as a very young child

Researchers also believe that a person's genetic make-up might play a role in developing anorexia.

Tell-Tale Signs

The most recognizable symptom of anorexia is severe weight loss. However, excessively thin arms and legs with little muscle tone or body fat, prominent cheek and **clavicle** bones, sunken eyes that have dark circles, brittle nails, and baggy clothes, are also indications that a person is suffering from anorexia. Some other tell-tale signs might be:

- not eating around other people
- obsessed with exercising, even if you're sick or hurt
- being petrified of gaining weight
- not menstruating for three months
- eating only very small amounts of food
- playing with food on the plate
- use of laxatives, diet pills, and diuretics
- depression, low self-esteem and self-worth
- feeling of having no control over your life
- tired all the time
- forgetful
- confused
- dry, blotchy, or yellow skin covered by soft hair
- always cold, even in warm weather
- weak with little body strength
- dry mouth

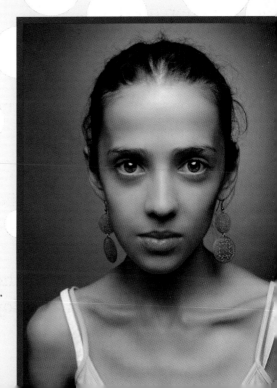

Among adolescent females, anorexia is the third most common **chronic** ailment. If not treated early, anorexia can have fatal consequences.

Body Breakdown

Anorexia, like other eating disorders, is usually triggered by a traumatic event such as divorce, death, or some form of physical or sexual abuse. The event leaves people feeling out of control. As a result, they use their bodies to gain back the control they believe they have lost.

People with AN are often depressed and feel little self-worth. They don't like their bodies. They don't like themselves.

Even though people with anorexia are extremely **undernourished**, they still think they are fat and will try to lose more weight to achieve what they believe is the perfect body weight.

The weight loss can become so severe that they have little or no fat left on their bodies. Yet, anorexia sufferers will still feel they need to lose more. Fat is essential for the body to function properly. Without fat, which is stored in cells, some vitamins can't be absorbed, and vital organs aren't protected from injury. Consequently, the various systems in the body begin to fail, including the **circulatory system**.

Although too much body fat can be unhealthy, your body still needs the fat stored in cells to function.

How Low Can You Go?

Anorexia can stop girls from menstruating. It can cause bones to become brittle and break easily. Kidneys can fail and the heart might beat abnormally.

Anorexia can also impact the circulatory system. People with anorexia can become anemic. This means that the blood is unable to carry enough oxygen to the organs, cells, and brain. As a result, they feel very tired. They cannot think clearly. Their emotional problems seem to get worse.

The more weight a person loses, the more serious the problem. While the solution might sound easy—just eat, right?—it is extremely complicated.

Anorexia nervosa is dangerous and can lead to death. The body can literally shut itself down.

Doctors consider anorexia nervosa the most dangerous of all eating disorders. Up to 10 percent of anorexic people die from medical complications. A person who undergoes successful treatment, however, still runs the risk of getting the condition later in life. That's why life-long treatment might be necessary to keep the illness in check.

By the Numbers

- One of the reasons boys are unlikely to seek help for an eating disorder is because boys believe only girls can suffer from the condition.
- Almost 14 percent of gay men suffer from bulimia and 20 percent from anorexia.

Source: National Association of Anorexia Nervosa and Associated Disorders

21

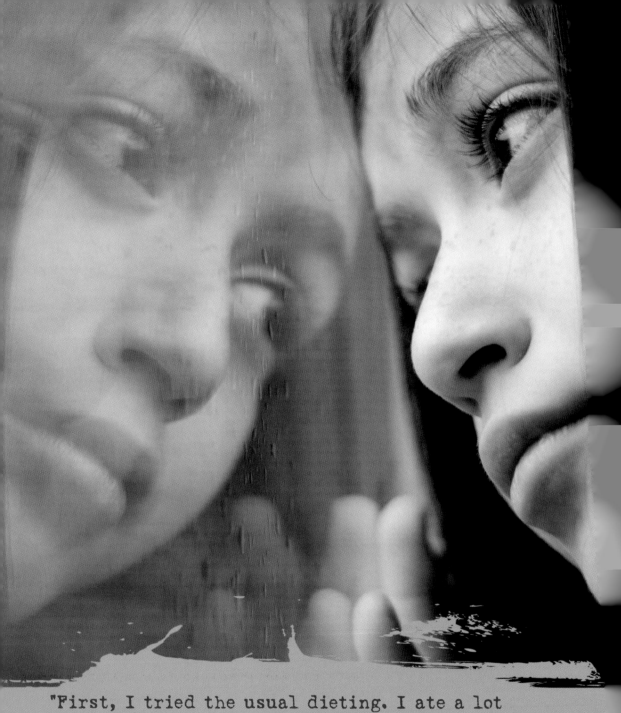

"First, I tried the usual dieting. I ate a lot
of canned soup. Nothing worked. I needed to do
something else. I wanted to become skinny and
sexy, just like the models in the magazines.
I forced myself to vomit." Tianna, aged 14.

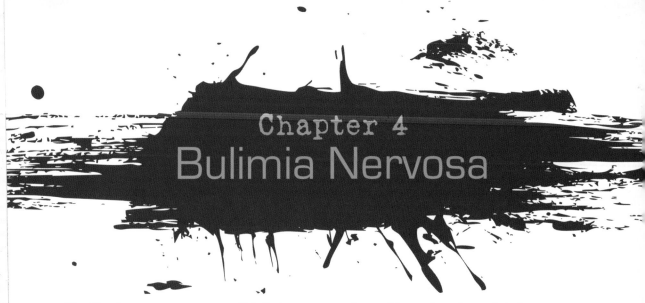

Chapter 4
Bulimia Nervosa

Bulimia nervosa, or BN, is an eating disorder in which a person consumes large amounts of food and then purges to avoid gaining weight. Like anorexia nervosa, bulimia is a mental disorder. The American Psychiatric Association classifies bulimics as those who binge, or engage in uncontrolled eating, and purging at least twice a week for three months.

Bulimics purge in a variety of ways. They use diuretics, laxatives, fasting, over-exercising, and self-induced vomiting. Bulimia can be triggered by any number of emotional or physical traumas including depression, a death in the family, a divorce or separation, or a physical assault.

Bulimics cannot stop themselves from eating. Yet, when they do eat, they'll binge on foods that are low in nutrition and high in calories. After binging, bulimics feel guilty for eating too much. They purge the food that they have ingested.

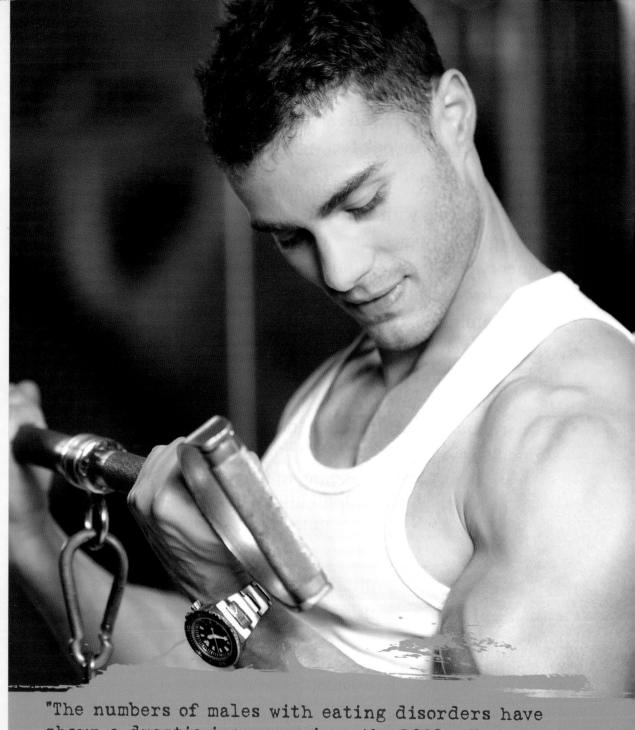

"The numbers of males with eating disorders have shown a drastic increase since the 1980s. How men look is becoming as important in the media as how young women look." Carla, clinical therapist.

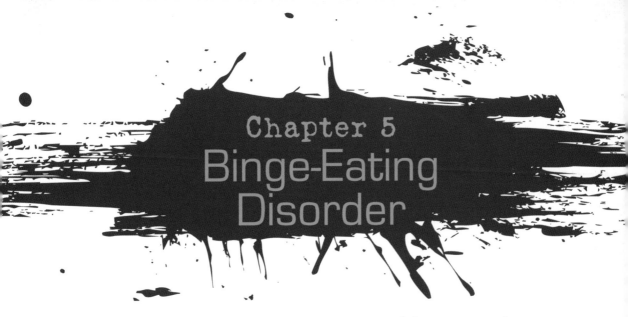

Chapter 5
Binge-Eating Disorder

Binge-eating disorder (BED) is a compulsive overeating disorder. Although BED is a lot like bulimia nervosa, there is no purging or excessive exercising involved. The affliction affects girls and boys, but is more often seen in females.

People who suffer from BED consume upwards of 15,000 calories during a binging session. Consider that an average, healthy adult male in his 30s needs between 2,500 and 3,000 calories per day.

Here are some characteristics of a binge eater:

- eating large amounts of food and promising never to do it again
- eating fast as they binge
- eating even after having a full meal
- expert at hoarding food, eating alone, and in secret

Researchers say your chances of having a binge-eating disorder are higher if there is someone in your family who had, or has one, too.

Mental Health Issues

Males and females who have BED tend to have impulsive personalities. In other words, they tend to act before thinking. There is also an association between BED and depression, low self-esteem, and low self-worth.

Often, those afflicted with BED have a history of substance abuse. In addition, many BED sufferers have high levels of stress. They find it hard to cope with negative emotions such as shame, self-loathing, boredom, worry, and anger. Such feelings can sometimes lead to suicidal thoughts.

Medical Problems

Physical complications associated with binge-eating disorder can be life-threatening. There is a high risk for teenagers to develop type 2 diabetes, high blood pressure, high cholesterol, heart disease, gallbladder disease, and other issues. BED is also linked to some types of cancer. Those with BED are also likely to suffer from joint and muscle pain, insomnia, menstruation problems, and headaches. If not treated, BED can be a lifelong problem.

Up and Down

So-called yo-yo dieting, or cyclical dieting, is one of the characteristics in the BED cycle. Yo-yo dieting is characterized by dieting or fasting, and then regaining the lost weight, if not more.

A University of California study of overweight women found that while yo-yo dieting quickly produces fast weight loss, subsequent dieting did not have the same results. In fact, the more a person dieted, the less weight they lost each time, and the harder it was to keep the pounds off.

Moreover, dieters put the weight on faster. The study recommended that no matter what a person weighs, it is important to strive for a healthy lifestyle. The key is to eat healthy foods in moderate amounts and exercise regularly.

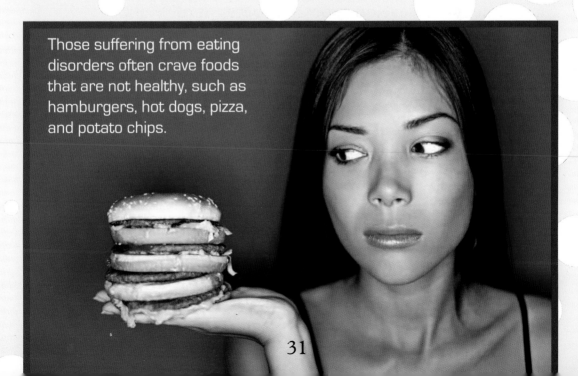

Those suffering from eating disorders often crave foods that are not healthy, such as hamburgers, hot dogs, pizza, and potato chips.

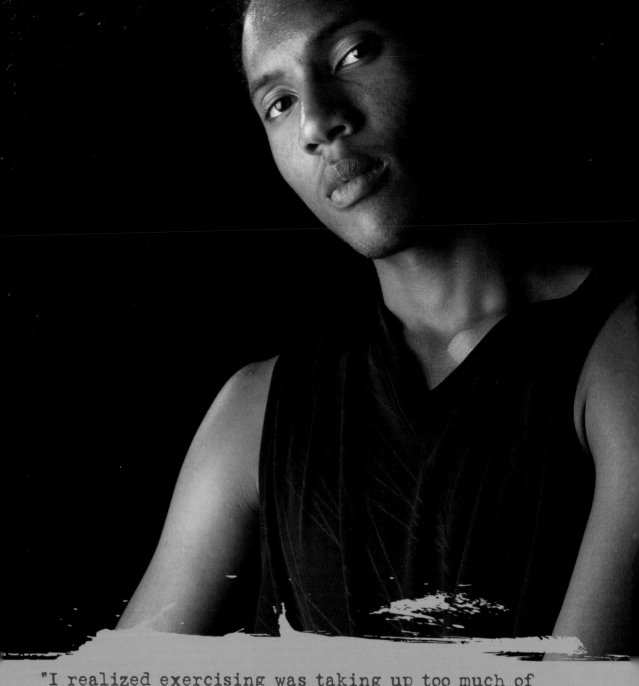

"I realized exercising was taking up too much of my life and making me too stressed out. That's when I started to think that there was something more wrong than just depression." Billy, aged 15.

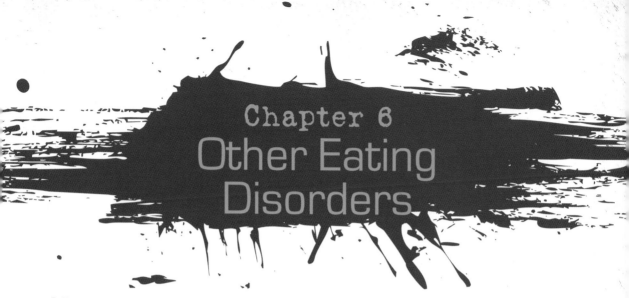

Chapter 6
Other Eating Disorders

Many people have heard of bulimia or anorexia. But, there are other, lesser-known eating disorders. Medical professionals often lump these conditions into a category called Eating Disorder Not Otherwise Named, or EDNON for short.

But there are other, lesser-known eating disorders. Eating disorders are complex. Many are a mix of anorexia, bulimia, and BED. Others, however, are completely unique.

Purging disorder (PD) is a common ED. It has attributes of bulimia nervosa. Those suffering from PD use diuretics, laxatives, enemas, and diet pills. Like bulimia, PD involves vomiting. The causes of the two are similar. According to some researchers, PD might actually be more common than both anorexia and bulimia.

Medical problems arising from PD depend on the method of purging. People who vomit often can damage their digestive tracts. If they use laxatives or enemas, they could suffer from severe diarrhea or **constipation**.

Night-Eating Syndrome (NES)

Night-eating syndrome is much more serious than just raiding the fridge at night. It affects people who suffer from anxiety and depression. People with NES will wake up in the morning not feeling hungry. They eat very little during the day. Once they go to bed, however, things change. They constantly wake up to eat.

Orthorexia Nervosa (ON)

Orthorexia nervosa is an obsession with eating foods of only the healthiest quality. The name comes from the Greek words "ortho," which means straight, and "orexia," which means appetite. While it is good to eat nutritious foods, people with orthorexia go overboard. If they eat anything else, they feel guilty and ashamed.

People with orthorexia are so obsessed with eating healthy that they limit their food intake to the point where they begin to starve themselves. Their bodies will eventually shut down. The kidneys will stop working, and the heart might begin to beat irregularly. Orthorexia can be fatal.

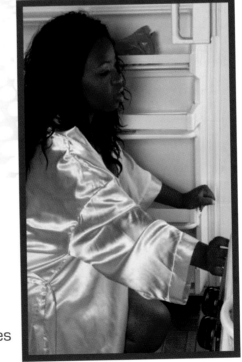

Eating nutritious meals is essential for good health, but when it becomes an obsession, it can be deadly.

Adonis Rising

The media often uses the term "manorexia" to describe male eating disorders. Although researchers believe 1 million males in the United States suffer from anorexia, most experts say this estimate is too low. In fact, the number might be as high as 1 in 4.

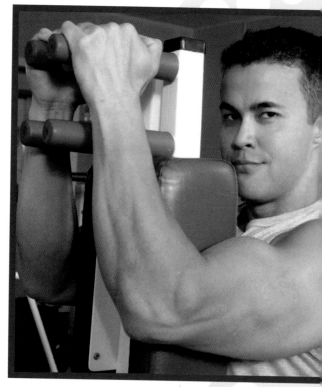

Some males with eating disorders will exercise excessively to achieve the "perfect body."

Athletic males have a higher risk of developing ED than non-athletic males. Guys who participate in gymnastics, running, figure skating, crew, and wrestling, have an even higher risk than other athletes. That's because these sports require leaner bodies. To develop muscles, males might resort to:

- eating only high-protein foods or supplements
- taking **ephedrine**
- using illegal **steroids**
- using food supplements to decrease appetite

A male preoccupied with not feeling muscular suffers from **muscle dysmorphia**, also known as the Adonis Complex.

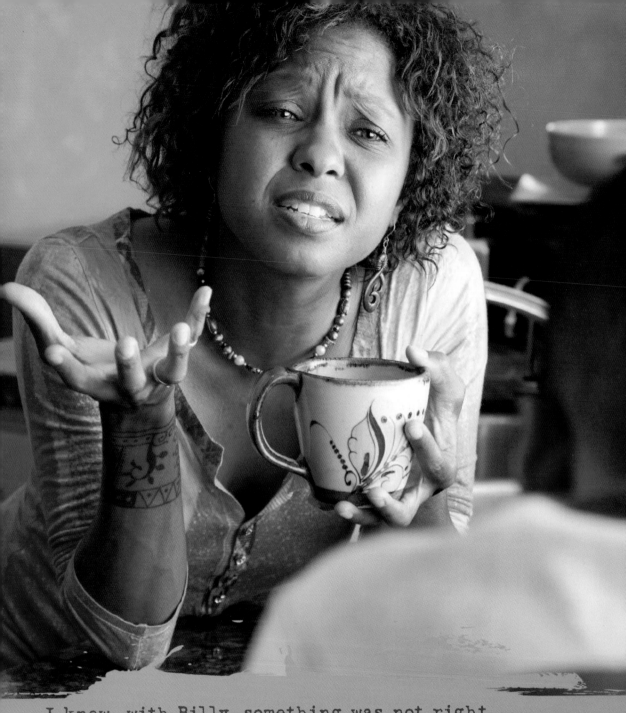

I knew, with Billy, something was not right...
He was cutting himself off from his friends, he
was fussy about his food, and he was losing weight
very quickly." Billy's mom.

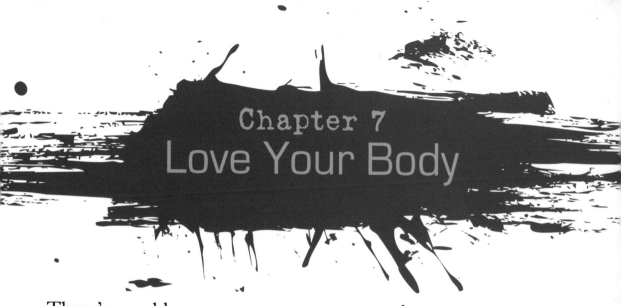

Chapter 7
Love Your Body

There's an old song your parents or grandparents might know. Its lyrics say "love the one you're with." Yet, you're the person you are with most of the time. Loving yourself is often difficult. At the end of the day, however, loving yourself is the only path to a healthy lifestyle.

Good self-esteem and a good body image can go a long way in how you feel about yourself. Self-esteem is how you think about yourself, and how you respect and value who you are. Body image plays an important role in self-esteem.

People suffering from eating disorders find it very difficult to love their bodies. They feel they are too fat, too big, not muscular enough, not strong enough. They believe their bodies lack the features of what desirable bodies are supposed to look like. Their self-worth is attached to this negative picture, which adds to their feelings of poor self-esteem.

Media Influences

Researchers believe that there are a number of factors that can cause people to have low self-esteem and negative self-images. The media, including TV, magazines, and the Internet, is often the biggest problem. The portrayal of Photoshopped, super-thin models, actresses, and muscle-bound jocks, makes many adolescents believe that this is what a normal body should look like.

The media's portrayal of the perfect body is so influential it can cause some people to develop eating disorders.

An interesting study of teenage girls on the South Pacific island of Fiji showed that the introduction of television in 1995 resulted in 15 percent of the girls inducing vomiting to lose weight. In addition, 29 percent were at risk of developing an eating disorder. Another 69 percent began dieting.

This may not seem unusual except that, in the Fijian culture, fat is considered beautiful. That all changed when television came to the island. The girls that were in the study said they wanted to be just like the thin actresses on their favorite shows.

By 2007, 45 percent of the girls said they used laxatives and had purged by vomiting. Also, 25 percent had considered suicide.

Bad Influences

Many people in the entertainment industry believe that having buff, thin bodies will help make them successful. Dance coaches often scold their students about their weight, forcing them to become thinner and more flexible.

In sports, coaches sometimes pressure athletes to become stronger and more muscular. Competition can often trigger an eating disorder.

Peer pressure can also cause an eating disorder. Smoking to keep from eating, fad diets, stimulants, diet pills, and exercising past exertion, all lead to unhealthy eating habits. A joke by a friend about looking fat, or a sibling's nasty comment can be enough to push someone with low self-esteem over the edge and into the pit of an ED.

What is a Healthy Body?

Maintaining a healthy body weight for your height by eating balanced and nutritious meals, along with moderate exercise and good mental health, goes a long way to boosting your self-esteem.

Keeping fit mentally is as important as good physical health. If you're feeling down, discouraged, or bad about yourself, don't wait for those feelings to get out of hand. Talk to a health professional, a school counselor, or trusted adult.

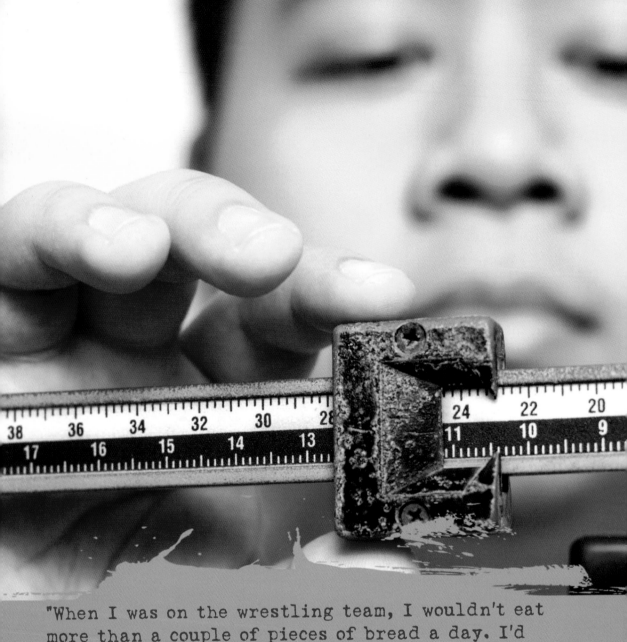

"When I was on the wrestling team, I wouldn't eat more than a couple of pieces of bread a day. I'd carry around a water bottle, even to class, just to spit in to lose water weight. I'd lose a couple [of] pounds a day that way so I could make my weight class." James, aged 21.

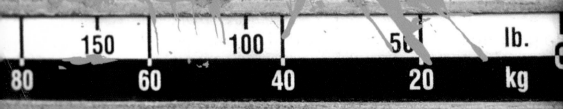

Chapter 8
Seeking Help

Doing something about an eating disorder can be difficult. First, you may not believe you are sick. Second, who can you trust? Third, what will happen to you if you tell someone?

Information is power. Before unhealthy eating habits, poor nutrition, and low-self esteem become too hard for you to handle, get help. If someone you know has an eating disorder, offer to help before the problem gets out of hand.

Educate yourself on eating disorders. Read everything you can on the subject. Find out where to get help. Talk to someone you trust. If you wish, look for organizations and agencies that will keep your information anonymous. It's important to get help as soon as possible. Reach out to a friend, the school nurse, or the principal. Help start a program that provides information about eating disorders in your school or community. Encourage a friend to talk and to get help before an eating disorder develops.

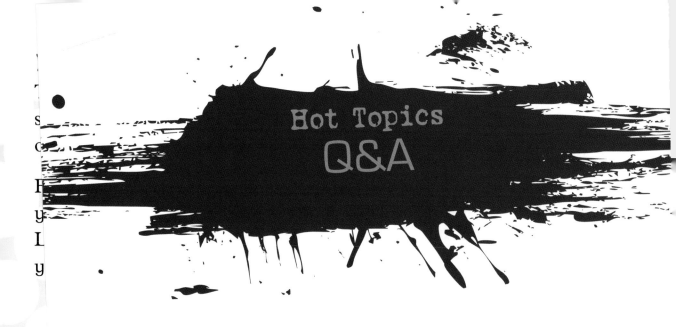

I don't want to eat all the time. Is that an eating disorder?

A: If your eating patterns are causing you to feel bad about yourself, you may want to talk to someone about it. Unusual eating patterns are not uncommon. They are called disordered eating. Seeking counseling can help you better understand the relationship you have with eating and answer your concerns.

Do eating disorders affect minorities?

A: Yes. Because only white females were studied by researchers for many years, it was thought that eating disorders were a predominantly middle-class, female, Caucasian condition. However, more recent studies using a broader base of people, including males, African Americans, Latinos, Asian Americans, and Native Americans, have given researchers a broader picture of how ED affects other groups.

My brother has ED. He's getting help, but it's so hard to watch him like this. Are there any programs for me and my family to help us get through this with him?

A: Talk to the healthcare professional that is helping your brother. Ask him or her to refer you and your family to a counselor, or to suggest a support group.

My friend is getting so skinny. But I'm not sure she has an eating disorder. She has lunch with me every day and eats as much as I do.

A: Even if your friend is eating, she is still becoming dangerously undernourished. Does your friend excuse herself to go to the bathroom right after she eats? Does she have bloodshot eyes, puffiness around her outer lips, or sunken cheeks? Does she brush her teeth a lot to get rid of bad breath? Your friend might be purging. Talk to her. Tell her you care and you are concerned about her well-being. And then talk to a trusted adult.

What type of research is being done to help people with ED?

A: Many different types of research are taking place—some of it with genetics, some with social issues, and others with psychological issues. ED is a complex web of different factors. There doesn't appear to be one simple answer that will solve the problem.

How do I find a good treatment program?

A: Your healthcare professional can recommend several places that can help with eating disorders. It's usually best to start with your family doctor.

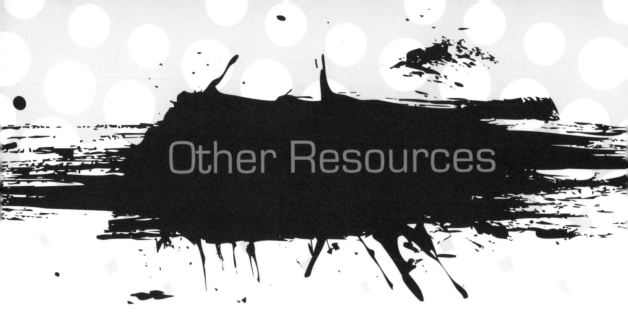

Other Resources

There is a lot of information available for people suffering from eating disorders and their families and friends. However, you might find that a lot of the information repeats itself. You might also notice that some of it is not reliable. Here are some sources you should find helpful. The Web sites contain information that is useful in the United States and Canada. Telephone numbers and referral services are good in either the United States or Canada, but not both. If you do call a number outside of your area, the helpline will probably refer you to a number inside your region.

In Canada

Eating Disorders Coalition of Waterloo Region
www.edacwr.com/
Good information on eating disorders, body image, and dieting.

Canadian Mental Health Association: Facts About Eating Disorders
www.cmha.ca/mental_health/facts-about-eating-disorders/
Describes eating disorders and how they are associated with mental health.

Mind Your Mind

www.MindYourMind.ca

A site designed specifically for young people. It deals with many topics and gives you a place to talk with others about your situation and your feelings.

In the United States

Eating Disorders Online: Eating Disorders in Men

www.eatingdisordersonline.com/eating-disorders-in-men

This site provides concise, relevant information and a meeting place for those seeking a path to recovery.

KidsHealth.org

www.kidshealth.org/

KidsHealth.org provides information about various health-related topics that you can trust.

Hotlines in the United States

Anorexia and Associate Disorders
1-847-831-3438

National Mental Health Association
1-800-969-6642

Hotlines in Canada

Mental Health Helpline
1-866-531-2600

National Eating Disorder Information Help Centre
1-866-633-4220

KidsHelpPhone.ca
1-800-668-6868

Glossary

avoidant personality disorder a mental illness which prevents people from interacting socially

calories Units of energy

carbohydrates One of three elements of food that contain starch and sugar used by the body for energy

chromosome A thread of DNA that carries genes

chronic Something that lasts for a long time

circulatory system The part of the body made up of the heart and blood vessels

clavicle The slender bone that runs from your chest bone to your shoulder bone

constipation Unable to have a bowel movement

dehydration Loss of body fluid

diuretic Drug that increases the output of urine

enema A procedure in which a liquid is injected into the rectum to remove its contents

ephedrine Drug used in the treatment of asthma and allergies

esophagus The tube that connects the mouth to the stomach

ethnicity A group with common culture, nationality and background

flatulence Gas produced from digestion in the intestines and passed from the rectum

genes Units of inherited characteristics that determine the characteristics of an individual, such as eye and hair color

genetically predisposed Genetic influences

hydrochloric acid The type of acid in the stomach used to break down food

Ipecac Syrup that induces vomiting

laxatives Drugs or substances that promote bowel movements

menstrual Relating to the monthly discharge of blood and other matter from the womb

muscle dysmorphia A mental illness in which a person becomes preoccupied with not being muscular enough

obesity Increased body weight caused by excessive fat accumulation

obsessive-compulsive Behavior that is uncontrollable and repetitive

oppositional defiant disorder A pattern of aggressive behavior to those in authority.

purging To remove or cleanse

steroids Synthetic hormones that can boost the body's ability to produce muscle

undernourished Poor nutrition due to unbalanced eating

Index